Diabetes

THINGS YOU SHOULD KNOW
(QUESTIONS AND ANSWERS)

By Rumi Michael Leigh

Introduction

I would like to thank and congratulate you for downloading this book, " *Diabetes, things you should know (questions and answers)*" series.

This book will help you understand, revise and have a good general knowledge and keywords of diabetes and how it affects the lives of people who suffer from diabetes.

Thanks again for downloading this book, I hope you enjoy it!

Chapter 1

1) What is diabetes?

- Diabetes is a disease which causes a high level of blood sugar.

2) Is diabetes a chronic disease?

- Yes, diabetes is a chronic disease.

3) What is the cure for diabetes?

- Actually, there is no cure for diabetes.

4) What is another name for blood sugar?

- Another name for blood sugar is blood glucose.

5) What is the normal value of blood sugar?

- The normal value of blood sugar is 100 to 125 mg/dl.

6) What is the cause of type 1 diabetes?

- Type 1 diabetes occurs when there is lack of insulin in the body.

7) What is the cause of type 2 diabetes?

- Type 2 diabetes occurs when there is resistance to insulin.

8) What is the function of insulin?

- Insulin regulates blood sugar. It brings down excessive blood sugar level.

9) How does glucose get into the cells?

- Glucose gets into the cells with the aid of insulin.

10) What is the function of glucose?

- Glucose feeds the cells.

Chapter 2

1) What is the main difference between type 1 and type 2 diabetes?

- The main difference between type 1 and type 2 diabetes is that in type 2 diabetes there is difficulty using insulin produced by the body and there is no production of insulin in type 1 diabetes.

2) What are the risk factors of type 1 diabetes?

- The risk factors of type 1 diabetes are hereditary, immune system damage, viral illness, etc.

3) At what age can type 1 diabetes occur?

- Type 1 diabetes can occur at any age.

4) In what kind of population is type 1 diabetes common?

- Type 1 diabetes is common in children population.

5) What is the main cause of type 1 diabetes?

- The main cause of type 1 diabetes is unknown.

6) Can type 1 diabetes be prevented?

- No, type 1 diabetes cannot be prevented.

7) How do the symptoms of type 1 diabetes develop?

- Symptoms of type 1 diabetes develop suddenly.

8) What kind of exercises is best for diabetic patients?

- The kind of exercises best for diabetic patients include aerobic exercises like walking, jogging, swimming, cardio exercises, etc.

9) When does hypoglycemia occur?

- Hypoglycemia occurs when there is a low level of blood sugar.

10) When does hyperglycemia occur?

- Hyperglycemia occurs when there is a high level of blood sugar.

Chapter 3

1) What is gestational diabetes?

- Gestational diabetes is diabetes caused by pregnancy.

2) What is the cause of gestational diabetes?

- The cause of gestational diabetes is that during pregnancy, the body of a woman becomes less sensitive to insulin.

3) What are the signs and symptoms of type 1 and type 2 diabetes?

- The signs and symptoms of type 1 and type 2 diabetes are frequent urination, fatigue, increased infections, increased thirst, etc.

4) What are the complications of diabetes?

- The complications of diabetes are heart diseases, stroke, kidney diseases, eye problems, dental diseases, etc.

5) What are the main risk factors of type 2 diabetes?

- The main risk factors of type 2 diabetes are inactivity, excess weight gain, age, high blood pressure, etc.

6) Why is weight gain a risk factor of type 2 diabetes?

-   Weight gain is a risk factor of type 2 diabetes because cells in the body reacts less to insulin due to increase in fatty tissue.

7) In what kind of population is type 2 diabetes common?

-   Type 2 diabetes is common in adult population.

8) Could younger adults and children develop type 2 diabetes?

-   Yes, younger adults and children could also develop type 2 diabetes.

9) What could be the main cause of type 2 diabetes in younger adults and children?

-   Increase in obesity rate could be the main cause of type 2 diabetes in younger adults and children.

10) Could type 2 diabetes be prevented?

-   Yes, type 2 diabetes could be prevented by having a healthy lifestyle.

Chapter 4

1) How do the symptoms of type 2 diabetes develop?

- Symptoms of type 2 diabetes develop slowly.

2) In type 2 diabetes, does the body produce insulin?

- Yes, in type 2 diabetes, the body produces insulin.

3) What are some of the causes of type 2 diabetes?

- Some of the causes of type 2 diabetes are obesity, lack of exercise and physical activities, etc.

4) Could type 2 diabetes be genetic?

- Yes, type 2 diabetes could be genetic.

5) What is the abbreviation DKA?

- Diabetic ketoacidosis.

6) What is diabetic ketoacidosis?

- Diabetic ketoacidosis is an emergency of diabetes mellitus.

7) Are ketones present in diabetic ketoacidosis?

\- Yes, ketones are present in diabetic ketoacidosis.

8) Is acidosis present in diabetic ketoacidosis?

\- Yes, acidosis is present in diabetic ketoacidosis.

9) Is hyperglycemia present in diabetic ketoacidosis?

\- Yes, hyperglycemia is present in diabetic ketoacidosis.

10) What are some treatments for diabetic ketoacidosis?

\- Some of the treatments for diabetic ketoacidosis are insulin, electrolytes, and IV fluids.

Chapter 5

1) Is insulin present in diabetic ketoacidosis?

- No, insulin is not present in diabetic ketoacidosis.

2) In what type of diabetes is diabetic ketoacidosis mainly found?

- Diabetic ketoacidosis is mainly found in type 1 diabetes.

3) What are the causes of diabetic ketoacidosis?

- The causes of diabetic ketoacidosis are stress, corticosteroids, undiagnosed diabetes, etc.

4) What are the signs and symptoms of diabetic ketoacidosis?

- The signs and symptoms of diabetic ketoacidosis are polydipsia, polyuria, nausea, vomiting, dehydration, fatigue, confusion, tachycardia, etc.

5) Does diabetic ketoacidosis happen gradually or suddenly?

- Diabetic ketoacidosis happens suddenly.

6) Is diabetic ketoacidosis more common with people with type 1 or type 2 diabetes?

- Diabetic ketoacidosis is more common with people with type 1 diabetes.

7) Should insulin always be injected in the same site?

- No, the injected site should be rotated/changed.

8) Why should the injected site of insulin be changed/rotated?

- The injected site of insulin should be changed/rotated in order to avoid tissue damage that could lead to absorption problems.

9) What is an insulin shock?

- An insulin shock relates to hypoglycemia.

Chapter 6

1) What is the abbreviation HHNS?

- Hyperosmolar Hyperglycemic Nonketotic Syndrome.

2) What is Hyperosmolar Hyperglycemic Nonketotic Syndrome?

- Hyperosmolar Hyperglycemic Nonketotic Syndrome is an emergency of diabetes mellitus.

3) Are ketones present in Hyperosmolar Hyperglycemic Nonketotic Syndrome?

- No, ketones are not present in Hyperosmolar Hyperglycemic Nonketotic Syndrome.

4) Is acidosis present in Hyperosmolar Hyperglycemic Nonketotic Syndrome?

- No, acidosis is not present in Hyperosmolar Hyperglycemic Nonketotic Syndrome.

5) Is hyperglycemia present in Hyperosmolar Hyperglycemic Nonketotic Syndrome?

- Yes, hyperglycemia is present in Hyperosmolar Hyperglycemic Nonketotic Syndrome but in a larger concentration.

6) What is the treatment for Hyperosmolar Hyperglycemic Nonketotic Syndrome?

- The treatment for Hyperosmolar Hyperglycemic Nonketotic Syndrome is hydration.

7) Is insulin present in Hyperosmolar Hyperglycemic Nonketotic Syndrome?

- Yes, insulin is present in Hyperosmolar Hyperglycemic Nonketotic Syndrome but in very little quantity.

8) Why is ketosis acidosis not present in Hyperosmolar Hyperglycemic Nonketotic Syndrome?

- Ketosis acidosis is not present in Hyperosmolar Hyperglycemic Nonketotic Syndrome because there is little quantity of insulin that prevents the body from metabolizing fat.

9) What is the cause of dehydration in Hyperosmolar Hyperglycemic Nonketotic Syndrome?

- The cause of dehydration in Hyperosmolar Hyperglycemic Nonketotic Syndrome is hyperosmolarity.

10) In what type of diabetes is Hyperosmolar Hyperglycemic Nonketotic Syndrome mainly found?

- Hyperosmolar Hyperglycemic Nonketotic Syndrome is mainly found in type 2 diabetes.

Chapter 7

1) Does Hyperosmolar Hyperglycemic Nonketotic Syndrome happen gradually or suddenly?

- Hyperosmolar Hyperglycemic Nonketotic Syndrome happens gradually.

2) Name an important cause of Hyperosmolar Hyperglycemic Nonketotic Syndrome.

- An important cause of Hyperosmolar Hyperglycemic Nonketotic Syndrome is infection.

3) What are the signs and symptoms of Hyperosmolar Hyperglycemic Nonketotic Syndrome?

- The signs and symptoms of Hyperosmolar Hyperglycemic Nonketotic Syndrome hyperglycemia is polydipsia, fatigue, fever, confusion, etc.

4) What is polydipsia?

- Polydipsia is a need of frequent drinking. It is having high thirst.

5) What causes polydipsia in relation to Hyperosmolar Hyperglycemic Nonketotic Syndrome?

- Polydipsia in relation to Hyperosmolar Hyperglycemic Nonketotic Syndrome is due to frequent urination.

6) What is a glucometer?

- A glucometer is a device used to check the glucose level in order to control blood sugar.

7) What is monogenic diabetes?

- Monogenic diabetes is diabetes that is mostly inherited and caused by gene mutation.

8) What is mutation?

- Mutation is a change in DNA sequence.

9) What is cystic fibrosis-related diabetes?

- Cystic fibrosis-related diabetes is when the body is not capable of producing sufficient insulin due to the scarring of the pancreas.

10) What is diabetic gastroparesis?

- Diabetic gastroparesis is when the movement of food slows down in the stomach due to nerve damage caused by diabetes.

Chapter 8

1) How is insulin injected?

- Insulin is injected subcutaneously.

2) Name the different types of categories of insulin.

- The different types of categories of insulin are rapid, short, intermediate and long.

3) Give examples of a rapid-acting insulin.

- Examples of rapid-acting insulin are Aspart, Glulisine, Lispro.

4) Give examples of a short-acting insulin.

- Examples of a short-acting insulin are Nivolin-R, Humulin-R, Regular insulin.

5) Give examples of an intermediate-acting insulin.

- Examples of an intermediate-acting insulin are NPH (isophane insulin), Humilin-N, Novolin-N.

6) Give examples of a long-acting insulin.

- Examples of a long-acting insulin are Levemir, Lantus, etc.

7) What is NPH insulin?

- NPH insulin is an intermediate-acting insulin.

8) What is a regular insulin?

- A regular insulin is a short-acting insulin.

9) What kind of insulin can be administered intravenously?

- Regular insulin can be administered intravenously.

10) Is a urine test enough to test for diabetes?

- No, a urine test is not enough to test for diabetes.

Chapter 9

1) What are beta blockers?

- Beta blockers are substances that decrease and slow down the work of the heart.

2) Do beta blockers cause hypoglycemia or hyperglycemia?

- Beta blockers cause hypoglycemia.

3) Does alcohol cause hypoglycemia or hyperglycemia?

- Alcohol causes hypoglycemia.

4) Does aspirin cause hypoglycemia or hyperglycemia?

- Aspirin causes hypoglycemia.

5) Do glucocorticoids cause hypoglycemia or hyperglycemia?

- Glucocorticoids cause hyperglycemia.

6) What are the signs of hypoglycemia?

- The signs of hypoglycemia are tachycardia, sweat, confusion, etc.

7) What is polyphagia?

\- Polyphagia is a frequent need to eat.

8) Which organ releases insulin?

\- The organ that releases insulin is the pancreas.

9) Which organ releases glucagon?

\- The organ that releases glucagon is the pancreas.

10) What is the function of glucagon?

\- Glucagon regulates blood sugar. It elevates blood sugar.

Chapter 10

1) What is HDL?

- High-density lipoprotein. HDL is known as good cholesterol.

2) Why is HDL considered to be a good cholesterol?

- HDL is considered to be good cholesterol because it removes bad cholesterol from the bloodstream.

3) What is LDL?

- Low-density lipoprotein. LDL is considered to be bad cholesterol.

4) Why is LDL considered to be bad cholesterol?

- LDL is considered to be bad cholesterol because LDL can surround and narrow the pathway of blood vessels by causing plaques.

5) What is cholesterol?

- Cholesterol is a fatty substance from the food we consume.

6) What organ produces cholesterol?

- The organ that produces cholesterol is the liver.

7) What are the functions of cholesterol?

- Cholesterol is used to produce bile, hormones and vitamin D.

8) What is bile?

- Bile is a fluid produced by the liver that helps with the digestion of fat and absorption in the intestinal tract. It removes bilirubin, etc.

9) What organ secretes bile?

- The liver is the organ that secretes bile.

10) Where is bile stored?

- Bile is stored in the gallbladder.

Chapter 11

1) What is the function of vitamin D?

- Vitamin D increases the intestinal absorption of calcium.

2) What is bilirubin?

- Bilirubin is a substance produced by the destruction of red blood cells.

3) Which cells specifically destroy the pancreatic Beta cells in type 1 diabetes?

- The cells that specifically destroy the pancreatic Beta cells in type 1 diabetes are the white blood cells.

4) Which organ is usually the first affected by low sugar levels in the bloodstream?

- The organ usually the first to be affected by low sugar levels in the bloodstream is the brain.

5) Why is the brain the first organ affected by low sugar levels in the blood?

- The brain is the first organ affected by low sugar levels in the blood because the brain needs a constant supply of blood to function properly and its main energy supply is glucose.

6) What happens when the brain doesn't receive enough glucose?

- When the brain doesn't receive enough glucose, it begins to malfunction and can cause severe complications.

7) What is a seizure?

- A seizure is an abnormal, uncontrolled and usually sudden disturbance of the electrical activity in the brain.

8) How are ketones formed?

- Ketones are formed when the body breaks down fat for energy.

9) Are ketones acidic or alkaline?

- Ketones are acidic.

10) Could diabetic ketoacidosis be a life-threatening complication?

- Yes, diabetic ketoacidosis could be a life-threatening complication.

Chapter 12

1) Is slow healing of wounds an indication of diabetes?

- Yes, the slow healing of wounds could be an indication of diabetes.

2) In what form is glucose stored in the liver?

- Glucose is stored in the liver in the form of glycogen.

3) Can the use of certain medications increase the risk of developing type 2 diabetes?

- Yes, the use of certain medications could increase the risk of developing type 2 diabetes.

4) Name some medications that could increase the risk of developing type 2 diabetes.

- Some medications that could increase the risk of developing type 2 diabetes are Thiazide diuretics, corticosteroids, etc.

5) What is hyperosmolarity?

- Hyperosmolarity is when blood becomes highly concentrated than normal.

6) What is the cause of hyperosmolarity?

- Hyperosmolarity is caused when water is pulled out of the body tissue into the bloodstream.

7) What are the effects of hyperosmolarity?

- The effects of hyperosmolarity are severe dehydration, seizures, etc.

Conclusion

Thank you again for downloading this book. I hope it has helped you in your journey to understanding diabetes and how it affects the people around you who suffer from it.

Please, if you enjoyed this book, I would like you to leave a review. It'd be appreciated.

Thank you.